30 DAY RESET

A spiritual guide for your health journey

LISA MCQUILLEN

THANK YOU

It is with a grateful heart that I want to say Thank You for coming along on this journey with me. My husband and I recently celebrated 4 years of marriage and also four years of infertility. I have the power to choose from which perspective I will view this journey and I'm choosing to see it through the lens of gratitude and blessings. I have seen God's hand in each step of the way and preparing us for something far greater. One area He has shown his blessings is in the community I have met along the way and the wisdom He has revealed to me through discovering Food Freedom! It is only because of this journey that you have this book in your hands and have made the choice to improve your wellness.

Mitch and I really got serious about choosing this lifestyle of clean eating and removing unnatural products from our home in February of 2018 as we looked for natural ways to overcome our infertility. I wanted to share with you some of the results we have been experiencing. I encourage you to share your results as well.

Both of us have experienced a balance in our Ph Levels, more energy, a more deep and restful sleep. We have seen our moods change for the better. We are both more present in the moment, more aware of our body and minds. We are no longer slaves to food and especially sugar, soda, alcohol. Mitch has lost 20 lbs., no longer snores at night, has gotten rid of a nagging cough and heel pain. I have not had a cold sore in 4 months, Praise the Lord. I am seeing progress in recovering from Adrenal Fatigue. I have been able to start running and working out again and feel energized by my workouts rather than fatigue. My digestion has improved, I no longer have foggy brain and am able to concentrate at work better. My skin is clearer, I handle stressful situations better and am able to be fully present in the moment and with conversations.

Whether you are looking to increase your energy, sleep better or shed a few pounds, you are in the right place! The Thirty Day Reset will be different than anything you have done before. This is not a "diet" rather a lifestyle change that will leave you changed from the inside out with a healthy relationship with food. You will be challenged mentally, physically and emotionally over the next 30 days, but you will also discover how amazing you can feel when you nourish your body with foods your Creator put here on this earth for you and cutting out foods that are most likely to cause issues.

You can do anything for 30 days.

ACKNOWLEDGMENTS

God – Thank you for this journey, your grace and wisdom as well as your patience in discovering your purposes for me.

"For I know the plans I have for you," declares the Lord, "plans to prosper you and not to harm you, plans to give you hope and a future" Jeremiah 29:11

"Have I not commanded you? Be strong and courageous. Do not be afraid; do not be discouraged, for the Lord your God will be with you wherever you go." Joshua 1:9

My sister LeeAnn, thank you for encouraging me to lead a group through my first 30 days and dreaming up wellness ideas with me on our morning runs!

Katie and Shantel for introducing me to Young Living in January of 2014 and opening my eyes to holistic wellness.

Jamie, you catapulted this idea off the ground with sharing your knowledge and wisdom with Mitch and I.

I'm grateful our paths have crossed Liz. Thank you for inspiring me, encouraging me to dream outside my comfort zone, challenging me and making this book a reality.

My husband Mitch and son Vince, thank you for putting up with my new ideas, trying new adventures with me, tasting my new recipes and most of all loving me for who I am.

And to YOU! Without You, none of this would be possible. Thank you for making the decision to invest in yourself and being a better you, Spiritually, Mentally, Physically, Emotionally from the inside out!

BEFORE WE BEGIN

PLANNING AND PREPARATION ARE VITAL

Please don't skip this step. If you wake up one morning and decide to start this challenge and haven't given this step any thought, you are setting yourself up to fail. I'm here to show you how to avoid this pitfall.

Here are a few important things to help ensure your own success:

Set the Stage for your family. Make sure they know you are doing this, especially your spouse. Tell them why. Maybe you want more energy to play with your kids. Maybe you want less joint pain. Maybe you want to shed a few pounds, which is not necessary the goal of The 30 Day Reset, but it can be an added bonus. Maybe you want to kick a craving. Maybe your why is even bigger, but I encourage you to write it down some place you can visually see it and be reminded of WHY you are doing this each and every day! Let's start by writing it down here:

_____

_____

_____

_____

Get Your House Ready. Go through your cupboards and pantry and tossing the junk food. If you want to save these items for family members not participating, dedicate a drawer, container or area that you will not be opening on a regular basis. Now is the time to do this while you are on fire and excited to start the program. This step is so important. If you feel bad about tossing food, give them to a neighbor or donate them to a local food bank.

Grocery Shop and Meal Planning. I'll be emailing you a list of compliant foods you can shop for.

The first few times you go grocery shopping it will take a longer to read labels so allow a little extra time or go when the grocery store is not as busy. I promise it gets easier. You may think it is more expensive to eat healthy, but my family has noticed we are saving money because we are not buying the expensive cereals, chips, prepackaged foods and alcohol. I meal plan on the weekend and grocery shop for exactly the items I need to make the meals I have planned out. I will also be emailing you a template for meal planning that will make it so easy and you will be less tempted to slip!

Check out Pinterest for meal ideas by searching for 30 Day Reset recipes or Google 30 Day Reset Recipes. I will also be sharing some of my favorites recipes that are kid and spouse approved. I will also be sharing with you on the go foods, eating out tips and emergency meals because we all know life happens.

You may be feeling anxious, overwhelmed, nervous, scared or maybe there is some excitement now that you've made the commitment. I want you to know that all of these feelings are normal, and you are not alone. I am here to support you, answer questions, encourage and pray for you on this journey. You will find yourself battling your fleshly desires, cravings, and emotions to give your body what it really deserves rather than a bunch of processed garbage.

In the beginning...

Are you familiar with the "creation story," detailing how God created everything we see?

On Day 1, light and dark.

On Day 2, the clouds and the ocean.

On Day 3, the Sun, Moon and Stars.

On Day 4, God created Plants, Trees, Fruits & Vegetables God said "Let the earth sprout vegetation plants yielding seed and fruit trees bearing fruit in which is their seed, each according to its kind, on the earth. And God saw that is was good.

On Day 5, Sea Creatures and Birds were created.

On Day 6, God created Man and Woman.

On Day 7, God rested.

> God created trees, fruits, plants and vegetables before He created man. Let that sink in for a second. Then God said to man, once he had created them "Behold, I have given you every plant yielding seed that is on the face of all the earth and every tree with seed in its fruit. You shall have them for food."

> Genesis 1:29-30.

Reflect on those words. God gave these things as a gift to man for food. When God created Man, He provided everything we needed, and He gave it to us in its best form with all the nutrients our bodies need to function optimally, the way He created us to function. Paving the way to fulfill his purpose. That's a pretty awesome God! Food has changed so much in the last 2000 years, but the way we are created to eat hasn't changed. This process helps us get back there.

Here is one last piece of truth I will leave you with today:

> "Do you not know that your bodies are temples of the Holy Spirit, who is in you, whom you have received from God? You are not your own; you were bought at a price. Therefore, honor God with your bodies."

> 1 Corinthians 6:19-20

Whether this is a spiritual journey for you or not, my prayer is that this is the beginning of you treating your body like a temple so that you may obtain physical, emotional and spiritual blessings. When those feelings of anxiousness, fear and worry creep in, try praying.

Take a few moments to write down how you have neglected to treat your body like a temple.

_____

_____

_____

_____

What physical, emotional and spiritual blessings are you hoping to gain from this journey?

_____

_____

_____

_____

Let's Talk Condiments.

This area can be as simple or complicated as you want it to be. Condiments are tricky because it is easy to sneak in additives to maintain color and shelf life. This is also an sneaky place to sneak in sugar and artificial sweeteners. The best way to avoid this is to make your own condiments, but don't judge yourself if isn't feasible at the moment. I want you to have this information for when you are ready.

I will be providing you with recipes for 30 Day Reset approved Ranch, Ketchup, Mayo and many others if you have the time and you want to make your own. If you don't have the time or maybe you are not a condiment connoisseur, there are 30 Day Reset approved condiments such as Tessemae and Primal Kitchen that you will soon discover. Coconut Milk and Coconut Aminos are also staples you will want to stock up on.

My advice is to take one thing at a time (don't try to do it all at once or you will feel overwhelmed), get comfortable with one item at a time, and your confidence will soar. Maybe try one new thing each day or week depending on your circumstances.

What condiment will you take first?

_____

_____

Here we go.

Make sure to get rested up, prepare your home and fill your refrigerator with lots of fresh produce.

Give Yourself 30 Days because YOU are worth it!

Take a deep breath, I know it seems like there is a lot to remember, but I promise you will get the hang of it quickly. You are doing this because YOU deserve it. Don't you dare let yourself think that this is going to be hard or you can't do it. Beating cancer is hard. Giving birth to a baby is hard. Losing a child is hard. Eating clean food that your body needs, was created to eat and deserve is not hard. Most likely you have faced greater difficulty. It's only 30 days and it is for you, the only physical body you will ever have in this lifetime. A Holy Temple. An amazing creation with purpose. A mother or father. A husband or wife. Someone whose why is to have more energy, loose a few pounds, beat infertility, wants to be able to keep up with their grandkids. Whatever your why is, remember it for the next 30 days. You never have to eat anything you don't want to eat. You are all big boys and girls. Learn to say no. It is always a choice to put food in your mouth. YOU WILL DO THIS!

DAY ONE

THE FIRST DAY OF THE JOURNEY

It's finally here. Your first day of 30 Day Reset. You are excited, you are ready to hit the ground running and tackle this first day with confidence. There is no question you are exactly where you need to be. It's no accident you are here, there is a reason, a purpose! You've got your pantry cleaned out, a refrigerator full of fresh produce, lunch packed, a meal plan ready for the week and a support group ready to cheer you on.

If you are planning to weigh yourself, this is the only time during the program it is recommended. Jump on the scale this morning, take some measurements and then hold off for 30 days. Focus on "Non-Scale Victories." Making it through day 1, eating a protein packed breakfast maybe for the first time in a while, drinking your coffee black, skipping your morning chocolate or your favorite beverage after work. Whatever it is, even if it may feel small, take the time to celebrate it and write it down below. It will be a compilation of lots of small victories that will get you through the next 30 days.

Day 1 Victory:

_____

_____

_____

_____

_____

_____

_____

_____

You are here for a reason. You are worth it. You are ready to gain control. You believe that honoring your body is what you are designed to do. You want another chance. You believe that this commitment to your own health and happiness will change everything. Today is Day One. You deserve freedom from food, we will do this together, one day at a time.

"I praise you because I am fearfully and wonderfully made; your works are wonderful, I know that full well."

Psalm 139:14

DAY TWO

THE HANGOVER

You may wake up this morning not feeling the way you thought you should after completing Day One. If you are feeling headache-y, foggy, week, slow, lightheaded and lethargic I reassure you, it's normal. Your body has begun the transition from running on carbs and sugar to becoming a fat-burning machine. Yep, you heard me, fat burning machine. The good news is it should only last a day or two.

When you wake up this morning, drink 16 ounces of water before you do anything else and be sure to drink plenty of water throughout the day. An easy rule of thumb is to drink half your body weight a day in water. If you add caffeine (coffee), add 8 oz. of water per cup you drink on top of half your body weight. So, if you weigh 150 pounds, you should drink 75 oz. of water and if you drink one 8 oz. cup of coffee you should drink 83 oz. of water.

Some of you may already be thinking, this is not what I signed up for, but be patient. Even the hard parts are part of the process. The sugar withdrawals, cravings and challenges that come with learning how to relate to good food in an entirely new way are evidence that something is changing. Every time you choose to keep going, distract your cravings and feed yourself with real foods, YOU WIN! Remember I said yesterday to celebrate small non-scale victories? This is what I am talking about.

What Non-Scale Victories did you experience today?

_____

_____

_____

_____

How many ounces of water did you drink today?

_____

_____

If you are feeling hungry, you may not be eating enough protein and healthy fats. No place in the The 30 Day Reset program does it say that you should be hungry. Be sure to eat the good stuff. Here are a few of my favorite emergency foods. What are yours?

Almond Butter (sugar free) with celery

Apples or banana with almond butter or a handful of nuts

Guacamole with carrots

A handful of nuts (with the exception of peanuts) mixed with raisins

If you are feeling tempted I'm here to tell you, even the greatest man to ever walk the earth was tempted, Jesus. Jesus had just spent forty days and forty nights fasting in the wilderness and was tempted by Satan. I can't imagine how Jesus was feeling. Tired, weak, hungry, delirious, cranky, slow (maybe similar to how you are feeling today). And what's the first thing He was tempted with? Food (bread). And here is Jesus' response:

"It is written, Man shall not live by bread alone, but by every word that comes from the mouth of God." He goes on to say, "Be gone, Satan!"

I encourage you, when you have times of temptation, cravings, weak moments, acknowledge them, pray and say NO, go away I am not giving in!

How were you tempted today and how did you react? How will you react differently the next time?

_____

_____

_____

_____

DAY THREE

EMERGENCY AND TRAVEL FOODS

Headed into the weekend and even if you don't have a busy weekend with lots of family activities on the calendar, these tips will come in handy. While these should be used sparingly and only in emergencies, please give yourself a little grace.

RX Bars – be sure to read the ingredients, not all are compliant
Lara Bars – be sure to read the ingredients, not all are compliant
Almond Butter with carrots, celery or apple – check ingredients to make sure there are no added sugars. We use Barney Butter (ordered off of Amazon)
Nuts – Pistachios, Almonds, Cashews, Walnuts, Sunflower seeds, etc. JUST NO PEANUTS. I love nuts mixed with raisins
Nick's Sticks – grass fed beef or turkey meat sticks with no sugar, no additives, no gluten and NON-GMO. You can purchase these at Hy-Vee and Amazon.
Raisins and Dates
La Croix Sparkling Water
Guacamole
Canned Tuna – watch ingredients. I found many contain soy
Shrimp
Hard Boiled Eggs
Canned Olives
Unsweetened applesauce

My husband travels almost every day for work. Prior to this lifestyle change he ate out when he traveled. His typical stop was the convenient store. (Ugh!) Needless to say, this was a huge adjustment for both of us and we had no idea how we were going to make this happen. When a dear friend shared this portable car food warmer with us, this lifestyle change became possible. Now, Mitch has a warm and healthy home cooked meal that he is able to take with him.

Extra bonus, is we are saving money because he is no longer eating expensive convenient store or fast food. This easily added up to $40-50 a week. You do the math. Here is a link to the portable food warmer for any of my traveling friends: https://www.amazon.com/YOUDirect-Electric-Heating-Lunch-Leak-Resistant/dp/B075NCZWZQ/ref=sr_1_1?ie=UTF8&qid=1524708356&sr=8-1&keywords=portable+car+food+warmer

What went well today?

_____

_____

What didn't go well today?

_____

_____

What will I do differently tomorrow?

_____

_____

Research shows it takes at least 30 days to change a habit.

"There is a time for everything, and a season for every activity under the heavens."

Ecclesiastes 3:1

.

DAY FOUR

SUGAR, IT'S MORE ADDICTIVE THAN COCAINE.

If you have begun reading labels and been out grocery shopping you will quickly realize sugar is hidden in almost everything. Why? Testing on mice proved sugar is more addictive than cocaine. Manufacturers want you to want to purchase and eat their food. They want it to be your daily or weekly habit. With all the choices out there, using sugar as a key product leaves you addicted and wanting to come back for more. Check out this article and YouTube video below:

https://www.huffingtonpost.com/connie-bennett/the-rats-who-preferred-su_b_712254.html

https://youtu.be/0EhwcSkShB8

Sugar comes in many different forms and names. Here is a list (not inclusive, but a good start):

Barley malt
Cane sugar (even if it says organic)
Corn Syrup
Evaporated cane juice
Fruit juice
Fructose
Galactose
Glucose
High fructose corn syrup

Lactose
Maltose
Maltodextrin
Mannitol
Sucrose
Sorbitol

Other sweeteners include coconut sugar, raw honey, date sugar, luo han guo (monk fruit), stevia, maple syrup, Xylitol. All of these are not approved by the 30 Day Reset program.

The Sugar Dragon.

If you haven't yet, you will soon experience the sugar dragon. Think back to a time when you purchased a package of Oreo cookies with the intention of having just one. Before you know it, you have scarfed down an entire row. How in the world does that happen? The sugar dragon is referred to as your brain's unrelenting demand for sugar, junk foods, or simple carbs. The more you feed it, the more fire it breathes and the stronger it gets. The only way to slay your Sugar Dragon is to starve it, which is why the 30 Day Reset allows for no added sugar, not some, not less, but none. Good news is, if you follow the 30 Day Reset Program your Sugar Dragon's fire breathing days are numbered!

Check in

Today's Non Scale Victories

Rate on a Scale of 1-10 with 1 being the worst and 10 being the best.

Energy

       Worst 1 2 3 4 5 6 7 8 9 10 Best

Sleep Quality

       Worst 1 2 3 4 5 6 7 8 9 10 Best

Cravings

       Worst 1 2 3 4 5 6 7 8 9 10 Best

What part of the day is most difficult for you?

_____

_____

What will you do tomorrow to overcome this difficulty?

_____

_____

Tips for slaying the sugar dragon:

Go for a brisk walk
Brush your teeth
Pray
Read a good book
Go outside
Play with your kids
Brew a cup of hot tea
Call a friend

I promise it won't hang around forever. It will go away soon!

DAY FIVE

CRAVINGS CAN LEAD TO COMPLAINING!

Congratulations! You made it through Day 4 and it's the end of the week! Give yourself some grace and a pat on the back. Some of you are still feeling tired, cranky, headaches and having some digestion issues. Others of you may already be starting to think clearer, have more energy and less bloated. However, you are feeling is normal. The amount of suck you feel is in direct correlation to the amount of junk you consumed before you started. Sorry soda drinkers, this makes the process harder for you.

Ticking Time Bomb.

Day 5 is known as TTB— the Ticking Time Bomb, because your brain doesn't like being told "no." Add other challenges like blood sugar dysregulation, digestive distress and whatever else you are maybe going through and it is no wonder you might be cranky. This too shall pass.

A few strategies to get through this moment in the process are to get plenty of sleep, add some Joy Essential oil over your heart or diffuse and choose a mindset of gratefulness. Choose a mindset of positive words like "I choose" or "I'm grateful for" rather than "I have to" or "I can't have that".

Pass on the complaining.

Whatever you do, don't let your cravings lead to complaining. Keep your end goal in sight. Remember me asking you to write down your WHY at the beginning of this journey and post it where you could see it every day? You need your WHY in front of you right now. Remember and focus on it. Your cravings and current circumstances are temporary.

There is a story in the bible about grumbling and complaining that I want to share with you. God had lead the Israelites out of slavery in Egypt and was leading them to the Promise Land (from slavery to freedom). However, this trip took several unexpected twists, turns, and challenges, and ended up taking longer than they expected (sounds familiar, right?). In fact, the Israelites ended up wandering in the wilderness forty years waiting to get to this beautiful place God had promised them. God provided for them every step of the way. He provided food (mana) for the 2 million people he was leading, every single day to quench their hunger, give them strength and sustain their bodies.

But they still grumbled and complained just like you and I do. The Israelites were focused on their circumstances rather than the end result of receiving God's gift of the Promise Land.

So, rather than focusing on your current circumstances, focus on the end, your WHY, count your blessings, be grateful and thank God for all the things HE has provided for you.

What's your why?

_____

_____

What are you grateful for today?

_____

_____

What positive words or phrases will you begin to say?

_____

_____

DAY SIX

HEAD TRASH.

I did it. This morning I ran 4 miles without stopping and I felt good, finishing stronger and faster than I thought I was capable. Some of you may be thinking I'm crazy to be so excited and others may be thinking it's no big deal, but for me this was huge. You see, I started running about 18 years ago. My first official race was the Chicago Marathon. I'm one of those gals that goes big or goes home. About 18 months ago, I was diagnosed with Adrenal Fatigue and I haven't run for the last six months. I have been recovering, learning how to support my body with food.

Why head trash?

You may be wondering why Head Trash is the title of today's motivation. When I was getting ready for my run this morning I started saying things in my head like, it's too cold, am I dressed warm enough, I can't do this, I have a sprained ankle, I'm not going to run as fast or long as I want. This my friends is Head Trash. We all have it and we all do it. Maybe some of you are struggling with Head Trash with this new way of eating. Telling yourself I can't do it, it's too hard, I don't have enough time to meal prep, cook and do all the dishes. I'm not saying some of this may not be true, but don't let the Head Trash in. Instead replace it with, I can do this, I choose to do this, I will make time today to go to the grocery store and stock my fridge with fresh fruits and vegetables, I will throw some burgers on the grill and use paper plates to save some time, the kitchen floor can be swept another day, I'm choosing to meal prep instead.

What head trash are you dealing with today?

_____

_____

_____

_____

What Non-Scale Victories dud you experience today?

_____

_____

_____

_____

How many ounces of water did you drink today?

_____

_____

_____

_____

DAY SEVEN

ONE WEEK OF W30!

Reaching the one-week mark of your journey may feel like you are surely past the worst of it. The anxiety, however, may not be receding. You may wonder if it's working. It's tempting to think, "I should check the scale to make sure it's working. Maybe you're even discouraged; "I thought I'd be further than this—shouldn't I be seeing more changes by now?" This is normal, given your history with dieting. It's been beaten into your head that for a diet to "work", you have to restrict, be hungry, and put your willpower to the test every second of every day. And this feels different and is different. You're eating delicious food. You're not starving (if you are, eat more and try adding more healthy fats to your meals). You are already seeing improvements. So instead of anxiety, decide that today is a day to feel hopeful.

The 30 Day Reset is not a diet, it's a reset. Taste buds, blood sugar regulation, hormones, digestion and your immune system are all returning to a healthy balance. You are resetting emotionally, too, learning a new language around food, changing your habits and creating awareness of how the foods you used to eat were impacting your self-confidence, motivation and quality of life.

The reset.

If you are having the urge to jump on the scale to see how far you've come, remember you are here for much more than weight loss. The scale won't reflect all the positive results you are seeing. You have so many other ways to measure your 30 Day Reset success (remember Non Scale Victories – NSVs). Are your rings, shirts or pants fitting better? Is your skin clearer, are your joints less swollen, is your nose less stuffy? Are you sleeping better? Here is a list of other NSVs you may be experiencing:

Mood, Emotion, Psychology

Happier	Less depression	More patient
Laugh more	Less anxious	Fewer mood swings
Handling stress better	Fewer cravings	Improved self esteem
Feeling in control of your food		

Physical (Outside)

Fewer blemishes	Flatter stomach	Less bloating
Improvement in skin color, rashes or patches	Longer, stronger nails	Less joint swelling
Stronger and thicker hair	Wedding ring fitting better	Clothing fitting better
Glowing skin		

Physical (Inside)

Less joint stiffness	Fewer PMS symptoms	Decreased stomach pain
Increased libido	Less constipation	Improved regularity
Less bloating and gas	Less sickness	Reduction in allergies
Fewer asthma attacks	Less acid reflux	Less heartburn
Less chronic pain	Less chronic fatigue	Less back pain
Improved blood pressure	Improved cholesterol	Improved blood sugar
Fewer headaches	Reduced or eliminated medications	Quicker recovery from illness

Food and Behavior

Healthier relationship with food	No longer using food as a reward	No longer a slave to sugar or carbs
No more binging	Able to eat mindfully	Learn how to read labels
Listens to your body	Identifies cravings vs. hunger	More nutrition in diet
More balanced meals	Learned how to cook	Learned how to use new spices
No longer afraid of healthy fats	Learn to enjoy and eat food slower	Drink more water
No more food guilt or shame	Healthy strategies to deal with cravings	

Brain Function

Think more clearly	Focus longer	Improved memory
Improved performance at job or school	Faster reaction times	Fewer ADD/ ADHD symptoms
More productive	Feeling more present or in the moment.	

Sleep

Better quality of sleep	Fall asleep faster	Less snoring
Feeling refreshed when you wake in the morning	Less night sweats	Difference in your dreams
Less sleep apnea	No longer need a sleep aid	

Energy

Higher energy levels	Energy levels are more stabilized	No afternoon nap
More energy at work or	Need less sugar or	No longer get cranky if

school	caffeine	you don't eat
More energy to play with your kids	More energy to exercise	

Sport, Exercise and Play

Start moving or exercising	Recover more quickly	More consistent with exercise
Can lift heavier things	Enjoying the outdoors more	Living a more balanced life
Trying new activities	Playing more with your kids or dog	Feel more athletic
Can exercise longer, harder or faster.		

Lifestyle and Social

More knowledge about nutrition	New healthy habits to teach your kids	Discovered new recipes
Spend less time and money at doctor's office	Taste delicious, healthy	Exploring other health goals
Met new friends	New cooking skills	Meal prep saves you time and you are more organized.

Community

Created and maximized your food	People come to you for health, food or lifestyle advice	Shop locally and eat seasonally.
Your kids have the best school lunch.	New lifestyle has brought your family closer.	Meal prep save

Check in

Today's Non Scale Victories

_____

_____

_____

_____

What NSVs are you experiencing?

_____

_____

_____

_____

DAY EIGHT

I JUST WANT TO SLEEP!

By this point, the train may have hit you. Are you tired, exhausted, just want to crawl in bed at 8:00 pm to sleep for 12 hours? You might be ready to nap at a moment's notice.

Your tiredness is no accident.

There is a science behind this experience. In the past your body was trained to run on sugar for fuel, thanks to the grains, added sugars and processed foods you had been eating. On the 30 Day Reset, no sugar, no carbs, no processed foods lifestyle, your body doesn't think it's getting any fuel. You feel like a car sputtering on empty. If you hang in there, however, the fat adoption process will begin in just a few days. It takes time for your body to recognize the healthy fats and vegetables available to consume. This explains why you are tired, maybe have headaches, fogginess, have cravings and are constantly hungry.

Food freedom.

The good news is you are a minimum of 6 days away from food freedom. The energized days are right around the corner. Listen to your body and get some extra, needed rest today. Crawl in bed at 8:00 or take a nap if you can. You are more likely to stick to your goal, not give into cravings and make better decisions if you are well rested. After all, it is Sunday. After creating the heavens and the earth, the water, the sun & moon, plants, animals and us, even God rested on the seventh day. God wants us to do the same. Rest and give Him praise and worship for all that he has done in your lives.

Change is difficult, and uncomfortable. We are creatures who like to be in control. Take hope because occasionally something happens that does the unthinkable and it makes us change what we want. This is what's going on in your body right now in relationship to food. I promise this change is good. You are only a few days away from seeing the long-term benefits. Give your body some much needed rest today.

What's happening on the inside.

Spiritually for Christians, change happens when Jesus grabs ahold of our hearts and makes us a new creation. Many of you are probably familiar with John 3:16 "For God so loved the world, that he gave his only Son, that whoever believes in him should not perish but have eternal life." Once a person's heart is captured by Jesus and they give their life to them, they are no longer in control. Jesus changes your priorities, the desires of your heart and what you want.

There is a man in the Bible whose name was Saul. Saul was the cream of the crop, highly educated and had a pristine job (The American Dream). He was working one day to deliver a letter to Damascus that would persecute and kill Christians. Saul took off by foot and suddenly was blinded by a light and the voice of the Lord spoke to him "Saul, Saul, why are you persecuting me". To make a long story short, Saul's name was changed to Paul and when he gained his vision back after three days, Paul was a changed man. He went from persecuting Christians, to laying his life on the line multiple times so that people would know who Jesus Christ is. He gave up everything.

Check in

What changes are you experiencing? What changes are you most looking forward to?

_____

_____

_____

_____

Today's Non Scale Victories

Rate on a Scale of 1-10 with 1 being the worst and 10 being the best.

Energy

       Worst 1 2 3 4 5 6 7 8 9 10 Best

Sleep Quality

       Worst 1 2 3 4 5 6 7 8 9 10 Best

Cravings

       Worst 1 2 3 4 5 6 7 8 9 10 Best

DAY NINE

HAPPY DAY 9!

Things are finally starting to feel like they're clicking—that is until your Sugar Dragon rears his ugly head. During the first week, it's actually easier to resist cravings; the program is exciting, and willpower is high. But rolling into week two (and not quite feeling the magic yet), you may start seeing temptation around every corner.

I've been preparing you for this for the last few days; reminding you of all the ways your 30 Day Reset is working so when the sugar starts calling, you'll be firm in your resolve. But don't panic if you're still having cravings. Your habits and emotions are still catching up with your new food choices, putting you in tough spots without allowing you the usual sweets and treats as crutches. It may feel like you're white-knuckling it past every temptation, but it will get easier as your taste buds change, blood sugar regulates, and you develop new healthy habits.

Handling the cravings.

How do I know if I'm hungry or just having a craving? It's not always easy to tell the difference, particularly in the heat of the moment, with temptation staring you in the face. Here are two methods to help you figure out whether your body just needs to eat something hearty and healthy, or it's just your Sugar Dragon breathing fire.

Halt.

HALT—stands for Hungry, Angry, Lonely, Tired.

The next time you're having a craving, stop and ask yourself, "Am I really hungry, or am I just angry, lonely or tired—or anxious, bored, frustrated, in pain?" You get the picture. If you can honestly assess that you're not really hungry and you can distract yourself for a few minutes to see you through. If the self-assessment helps you realize you really are hungry, then eat a full meal or a mini-meal to tide you over.

The steamed fish and broccoli question.

This next trick is a bit simpler, but brutally effective. Just ask yourself, "Am I hungry enough to eat steamed fish and broccoli right now?" (or hard-boiled eggs and guacamole, or plain roasted chicken with carrot sticks.) If the answer is, "No, but I'd eat an RxBar or some grapes, " you are just experiencing a craving, so distract yourself accordingly. However, if the answer is "Yes" then you really are hungry. Eat a small meal of protein and vegetables!

The 30 Day Reset Egg Burrito

It's important to fuel your body with a healthy protein first thing in the morning. Eggs are my go-to for a simple, nutritious and protein packed breakfast. Not only does protein wake your body up, but it is an excellent source of energy that takes longer to digest and therefore will leave your body feeling fuel longer. This is the opposite of a breakfast full of sugar and processed carbs, which leave you feeling good for a short period of time. Then you are left to crash and burn, feeling tired, hungry and like a failure.

This Whole 30 compliant Breakfast Burrito is delicious, gluten free, dairy-free, sugar free and a guilt free way to start your day!

Ingredients

> 2 slices of Whole 30 compliant bacon
> 1/2 Avocado
> 1 handful of spinach
> 3 large eggs
> 2 tablespoons coconut oil
> 2 tablespoons unsweetened almond milk
> Salt and Pepper to taste

> Optional

> You can always add your favorite veggies to any burrito to make it your own. Onions, Peppers, Tomatoes, Mushrooms. Get creative and be original.

Instructions

First, place coconut oil in a 10-inch non stick frying pan and heat on medium. I use a copper pan and it works great.

While the oil is heating whisk together 3 eggs and unsweetened almond milk in a bowl.

Add your favorite vegetables (onions, peppers, tomatoes, mushrooms, etc.) and season with salt and pepper.

Pour eggs into the pan and allow to cook without touching until they start to set up. Gently lift up the edges of the egg formation and tilt the pan so the remaining running egg mixture runs to the pan and begins cooking.

Continue moving around the sides of the pan until the majority of the egg is set. Flip the egg formation over and cook on the other side.

Top with bacon, spinach, avocado, salsa.

This burrito would go perfect with a side of hash browns and a piece of fruit for a Whole 30 compliant breakfast, lunch or dinner!

What's your favorite way to make eggs?

_____

_____

_____

_____

It's not a sprint, it is a marathon.

"Do you not know that in a race all the runners run, but only one gets a prize? Run in such a way as to get the prize. Everyone who competes in the games goes into strict training. They do it to get a crown that will not last, but we do it to get a crown that will last forever. Therefore, I do not run like someone running aimlessly; I do not fight like a boxer beating the air. No, I strike a blow to my body and make it my slave so that after I have preached to others, I myself will not be disqualified for the prize."

1 Corinthians 9:24-27

DAY TEN

DON'T QUIT

Warning: these next couple days can be the toughest days. You are most likely to quit and waste all your hard work. The newness of the program has worn off. You've experience lots of the negatives but have yet to see the "magic". You are asking yourself, "Will the results really be as good as the say?" You are cranky, hungry and tired.

Take a deep breath.

This is where you really start to experience the psychological power of your prior food choices and habits. Your brain is throwing a tantrum because it senses that this time, you are serious about making changes and quick-and-easy rewards will no longer be a regular occurrence.

Your brain is demanding a reward, because you deserve it, right? We are a culture that rewards with food and you've been a product of it for 20, 30, 40 or 50 years. When was the last time a cupcake ever made you feel accomplished, comforted or confident? It's time to find another way to meet that need, because you deserve more than the craving-overconsumption-guilt-stress cycle you've been stuck in. Remember your WHY? You need to focus on your WHY these next couple days.

What's your long term, most significant reason for completing these next 20 days?

_____

_____

_____

Dig in for success.

It's time to reach out for support. Others around you can see changes that you may be overlooking. If you are hungry, eat more healthy fats and protein. They take longer for your body to break down and digest, so they will keep you full longer. Treat yourself with a new kitchen gadget that will make this journey easier, maybe a new cookbook, yoga mat, pedicure, massage, just something other than food. If you need support and encouragement, private message me. I would love to talk with you, encourage you and pray with you.

How will you reward yourself rather than using food?

_____

_____

_____

_____

DAY ELEVEN

GROWTH

You've been go-go-go on your 30 Day Reset; planning meals, prepping food and doing three days' worth of dishes every night. You are starting to form better habits, getting more comfortable with what is compliant and what is not. You are finally reaching the peak of the roller coaster. You're not over the hump yet, but you are starting to see it—small signs of growth.

Envision a tiny seed, not yet sprouted. It is miraculous that one tiny seed eventually blossoms into a beautiful plant producing fruit and vegetables. It takes days of nurturing with the proper soil, sunlight, water and temperature. It appears as if nothing is happening for days until "suddenly," overnight a sprout appears. It may seem small, but it is evidence of growth. This reminds me a lot of our 30 Day Reset Journey. After several days of persistence, meal prepping, nurturing your bodies with the right foods, the proper amount of rest, determination and discipline, some of you may be starting to see signs of small growth. For others, this growth is waiting to sprout out of the soil you have been nurturing, but it is there even if you can't see it.

This also reminds me of the Parable of the Mustard Seed:

> "The kingdom of heaven is like a grain of mustard seed that a man took and sowed in his field. It is the smallest of all seeds, but when it has grown it is larger than all the garden plants and becomes a tree, so that the birds of the air come and make nests in its branches."

Matthew 13:31-33

Jesus goes on to say in Mathew 17:20 "For I truly say to you, if you have faith like a grain of mustard seed, you will say to this mountain, "move from here to there,' and it will move, and nothing will be impossible for you."

What's your Mountain? Do you have Faith?

_____

_____

_____

_____

Whether you realize it or not, you are living by faith every day. Choosing to do the 30 Day Reset took faith that you will get results.

God takes the tiniest bit of faith we have and makes it grow into something big when we act on it. The Bible says that "God has dealt to each one a measure of faith." Romans 12:3. We already have some faith to start with. When we step out in that faith, God increase our faith.

We have no idea what great things God wants to do through us if we would just step out in faith when He asks us to.

Where are you seeing growth?

_____

_____

_____

_____

How can you step out in faith today? Maybe it's trying a new vegetable, a new recipe, maybe it's giving someone a compliment or just saying thank you.

_____

_____

_____

_____

DAY TWELVE

YOUR TASTE BUDS ARE CHANGING.

It's day 12 and you're feeling the downhill momentum. You wake up strangely happy, cautiously optimistic and feeling pretty darn good. Your "Tiger Blood" hasn't fully kicked in yet, you may still have some cravings, and the dishes just won't end. Yet, you're tossing your 30 Day Reset lunches together effortlessly; someone offered you a donut at work and you didn't think twice before saying, "No, thank you' and that orange you just ate….is this what an orange is supposed to taste like? It's so pure and sweet—what is happening to you?

The 30 Day Reset is happening. Your taste buds are changing, your blood sugar is better regulated, your hormones are doing their job and your immune system is calming down, Everything is starting to work the way God intended, so your body is sending you all the right signals. It's not ALL sunshine and rainbows from this point, but if this is you today, throw your hands in the air and enjoy the ride.

So, what has changed?

You are starting to notice more flavor in whole foods, as you bite into a fresh strawberry or banana it tastes different. You notice the texture and it's sweeter than it used to be. Those sweet potatoes or sautéed vegetables have entirely new flavors. You are learning to become more confident with spices and their ability to change the flavor of your dish. This reinforces your new, healthy habits, and may lead you to prefer the natural sweetness of a strawberry over the artificial, sickly-sweet flavors of your beloved donuts. In fact, post 30 Day Reset, you may find your old favorite processed treats aren't so delicious anymore.

My hubby has put this to the test. Anyone that knows him, is aware that his most favorite food in the world is chips. He is known as a chip connoisseur. Before we changed our lifestyle, he would tell you that if he was left on this planet with one food, he would want it to be chips. After we had been on our new lifestyle for about 10 weeks, he tried a handful of Kettle Cooked Potato chips and found them disgusting. This is huge and evidence that The 30 Day Reset works. Please don't run out and put this to the test yet. Take my word for it and soon enough, you will have completed this journey and can test it yourself.

In order to complete the 30 Day Reset by the book, you first need to believe you can. Getting rid of the head trash that you can't do this and replacing it with self-affirmation, encouragement and positive thinking is instrumental in shifting your mindset. Boosting your belief that you can (and will) finish strong and successfully will change the next 18 days. If you are looking for a great read check out the book, **Conscientious Languages,** to learn more about this idea of we become what we think. You've got 12 days of 30 Day Reset behind you, you are going to finish strong, this will change your life. Embrace it. I knew you could do this from the start and now you do too.

What will you say to yourself different to affirm your success in the next 18 days?

_____

_____

_____

_____

Check in.

Today's Non Scale Victories

Rate on a Scale of 1-10 with 1 being the worst and 10 being the best.

Energy

Worst   1   2   3   4   5   6   7   8   9   10   Best

Sleep Quality

Worst   1   2   3   4   5   6   7   8   9   10   Best

Cravings

Worst   1   2   3   4   5   6   7   8   9   10   Best

DAY THIRTEEN

LET'S TALK HEALTHY FATS.

Day 13 is generally a mixed bag. Many of you are starting to feel the magic, sleeping better, energy more consistent, and cravings mostly under control. Many of you are tired—either still tired or back to being tired. You were feeling good, and now you're not as energetic, or your energy fades as the day goes on. This is really common and often means you're not eating enough, yep, I'm going to say it, FAT! You need healthy fats to flip the switch. What switch am I talking about?

Why do I need fat?

Magical things happen when you start eating real, nutrient dense, satiating food. It may feel like you are eating a lot, but during this process, the switch happens when your body learns to burn fat as fuel (rather than sugar/carbs) and reconnects you with "hungry" and "full" signals and ditches the sugar cravings So if you are still feeling tired or hungry, increase your healthy fats. For some, this goes against everything you have ever learned, but it works.

Here is a list of healthy fats:

> Almonds
> Almond butter
> Almond milk (unsweetened)
> Cashews
> Coconut oil
> Olive oil
> Pecans
> Sunflower seeds

Pumpkin seeds

Chia seeds

Flaxseed

Sesame seed oil

Ghee

Olives.

If you are pregnant or nursing, have an active job, work long days or exercise a lot, three meals a day may not be enough for you. And that's okay. Simply be sure to leave at least 3-4 hours between meals to allow your hormones do their job.

Tip: On a personal note, we learned on our journey that we were eating too many potatoes. Hash browns for breakfast and some type of potato for dinner. We weren't seeing the waistline changes like we were hoping for. We didn't change the amount of food we were eating, but replaced the potatoes with healthy fats and lots of vegetables. It worked for us!

How will you adjust your fat intake?

_____

_____

_____

_____

What will you do different tomorrow?

_____

_____

_____

_____

Is there a new healthy fat from the list above you are going to try?

_____

_____

_____

_____

DAY FOURTEEN

TWO WEEKS.

You're sleeping better, your skin is clearer, you're more self-confident, you no longer need a nap at 1 pm, your pants have extra room, temptations are easier to decline, and managing your meal planning and emergency food feels, dare we say it—feels nearly effortless. On the flip side, food boredom may be setting in, you're still feeling stressed when socializing and you may be trying to boost your energy by eating more.

For some of you, every morning brings new NSVs. For others, you're definitely noticing improvements, but still struggle with digestions, bloating, energy or other symptoms. Take heart-the benefits you are seeing are a clear sign that you are moving in the right direction. There is a reason this is not called WHOLE14, hang tight.

Small changes make a big difference.

Seriously, can we talk about all the dishes? Maybe it's time to make some changes.

Here are a few tips:

> If you are doing all the cooking, have your husband or kids do the clean-up.
>
> Have the kids empty the dishwasher and refill when they get home from school.
>
> Prep all your ingredients before you start.
>
> Use one big cutting board for all your veggies rather than multiple small ones.
>
> Use the same pan to cook your entire meal, or better yet, use the grill.

Paper plates are just sometimes a must.

Have a sink full of hot soapy dishwater (of course with Young Living thieves dish soap). As your onions are sautéing in the pan or in-be-tween flipping the meat on the grill, wash a couple dishes, wipe off the counter, etc.

Shift other responsibilities (if you can) to another family member. It's a great time to teach your kids responsibility and why you have chosen a healthier path for you and your family. If you don't have others to help out, maybe it's time to reprioritize.

What can you let go of or what's maybe not as important as giving your body the nutrition it needs and deserves?

Decrease your stress.

A University of California study measuring stress hormone levels in 30 couples found that people who describe their home environment as "chaotic" or "messy" had higher levels of cortisol (stress hormone) when measured at various points throughout the day (this is so me, but I'm working on getting better with this).

Note: chronically high levels of cortisol wreak havoc in the body, promoting sleeplessness, inflammation, and weight gain, so keeping stress levels downs is important! A tidy kitchen could mean a calmer, more confident, happier 30 Day Reset kitchen. Before you go to bed spend five minutes tidying up your kitchen. Waking up in the morning to a clean organized kitchen could help your mindset for the day!

What responsibilities can you shift or release?

_____

_____

_____

_____

How can you get your family involved with helping and being a part of this journey

_____

_____

_____

_____

Take 5 minutes to tidy up your kitchen tonight before you go to bed. Place frozen meat in the fridge so it is ready to go for tomorrow. Use the crockpot to cut down on the dishes.

Here is a list of some of my favorite help kitchen gadgets:

> Large cutting board
> Cast Iron Skillet
> Ninja Blender
> Food Processor and Spiralizer
> Air Fryer
> Crockpot
> Instapot
> Garlic press
> Small glass storage containers for storing leftovers
> Extra measuring cups and spoons
> Don't forget paper plates!

DAY FIFTEEN

YOU ARE HALFWAY THERE.

Today you have conquered or survived two 30 Day Reset weekends and you're finding it easier to say no to temptations and navigate social situations. Take some time for a Non Scale Victory lap as your taste buds continue to change and that strawberry or sweet potato you just ate was thoroughly enjoyable.

Don't use a shovel.

It's time to address one of my weaknesses: the battle between mindful eating or shoveling it down the hatch. Everyone in my house will hands down agree that I am the world's fastest eater. I wish I could take time to enjoy my food and savory each bite rather than eating and rushing on to the next thing. I am working on this!

Most Americans eat way too fast and don't chew their food properly. As a result, they take in extra calories, ultimately resulting in weight gain. It takes approximately twenty minutes from the time you start eating for your brain to send out signals of fullness. When you slow down, savor a meal, pay attention to tastes and texture and appreciate each mindful bite, you leave the table feeling good in your soul, no matter what you ate.

Slowing down your eating also helps the digestion process. Digestion starts in the mouth, so large bites that are inadequately chewed will be more difficult for your stomach to process. Different places I checked out said you should chew your food 30-40 times before swallowing. Food that isn't properly broken down can lead to indigestion and other potential GI problems. Who wants to deal with that?

Social Outings.

Perhaps you feel you have to be a hermit to succeed in this process. You can't go anywhere because you're not sure if the food will be 30 Day Reset compliant. Declining social invitations can be a good strategy in the beginning, but you eventually you need to build confidence in your health-minded choices in any setting, including business lunches, bridal showers, birthday parties, barbeques, weddings, or anything you can dream up.

I have a few tips to help you along the way:

Plan and Prep.

Eat before you go, research the menu ahead of time, bring your own dressing, pack emergency foods.

Be confident.

Be totally confident in your restaurant order. "I'll have the burger, no bun, no cheese and instead of fries, can I have mixed vegetables, please?" The bigger the deal you make out your dietary choices, the more you will call attention to them, so nonchalantly place your order and return to the conversation.

Do socialize.

You can bond with co-workers at happy hour just as effectively with sparkling water in your glass, and you may even enjoy it more (especially the next morning). Be polite and say "No, thank you," with confidence and a smile! Social encounters are not about the food on your plate—they are about the people you are with, the relationships you are building, the connections you make and the memories you create.

Bring a 30 Day Reset compliant dish to share.

Attending your next BBQ or Birthday gathering? Bring one of your favorite dishes to share. People are noticing your clearer skin, energy, confidence and just a healthier glow about you when you enter the room. Share your experience. I bet someone will even ask for the recipe!

What social event do you have coming up on the calendar and what will you do to prepare

_____

_____

_____

_____

What go to meal or side dish have you discover that you are ready to share with others

_____

_____

_____

_____

How will you be more mindful of slowing down and chewing your food today

_____

_____

_____

_____

DAY SIXTEEN

CHOOSE JOY.

It's day 16, some of you may be thinking "I'm on the downhill slide" others may be thinking, "this 30 Day Reset thing is not so bad, maybe I could make this a new lifestyle with a few exceptions" Changes are happening, and you should embrace them with JOY!

Here is a reminder of God's provision and love for us in providing food:

> "You cause the grass to grow for the livestock and plants for man to cultivate, that he may bring forth food from the earth and wine to gladden the heart of man, oil to make his face shine and bread to strengthen man's heart."

> Psalm 104:14-15

I know what some of you may be thinking, Wine? Bread? Yep, God provided those for our enjoyment too, but not until we get through a few more days. And I'm pretty confident wine and bread were made entirely differently than we make them today.

Let's talk beverages.

There is an overabundance of beverages out there to choose from. Water is always best, and you should be drinking at least ½ your body weight in ounces of water each day. If you aren't fulfilling this requirement, now is a time to refocus. You've been so consumed with finding compliant recipes, doing dishes and not giving into your Sugar Dragon the past 15 days. As things start to get a little easier, maybe now is the time to start focusing on other healthy habits.

Other Beverages:

Organic Coffee.

Organic is less acidic than non-organic.

Water.

Add a few drops of your favorite vitality oil (Peppermint, tangerine, lemon, orange, lime).

Green Tea or Matcha Tea.

Matcha Tea is very popular right now. It is different than regular green tea for a few reasons: One serving of matcha tea is the nutritional equivalent of 10 cups of regularly brewed green tea. When you drink matcha you ingest the entire leaf and receive 100% of the nutrients of the leaf. Matcha powdered green tea has 137 times more antioxidants than regularly brewed green tea. It also boosts metabolism, is a natural detox, calms the mind and relaxes the body, is rich in fiber, chlorophyll and vitamins, enhances mood and concentration, provides vitamin C, selenium, chromium, zinc and magnesium, can help lower cholesterol and blood sugar.

LaCroix. Carbonated sparkling water
Unsweetened Almond Milk. Read ingredients
Unsweetened Coconut Water. Read ingredients
Club Soda
Kombucha. Check the ingredients especially for added sugars
Mineral Water
Seltzer Water
Sparkling Water. Read your labels
Vegetable Juices
Water Kefir
What beverage have you ditched because of the added ingredients? What new beverage are you enjoying

Check in.

Today's Non Scale Victories

Rate on a Scale of 1-10 with 1 being the worst and 10 being the best.

Energy

        Worst   1   2   3   4   5   6   7   8   9   10   Best

Sleep Quality

        Worst   1   2   3   4   5   6   7   8   9   10   Best

Cravings

        Worst   1   2   3   4   5   6   7   8   9   10   Best

DAY SEVENTEEN

TIGER BLOOD.

It's Day 17, and for most 30 Day Reseters, that spells "Tiger Blood." According to Melissa Hartwig's Whole30 Day by Day, the phrase Tiger Blood originated with Charlie Sheen, but we adopted it to describe the consistent energy, happy mood, rockin' self-confidence and NSVs you're feeling at this point in your 30 Day Reset Journey. Now don't stress if this isn't you yet. Not everyone experiences Tiger Blood on exactly the same day. There are other factors, age, health history, past dietary habits and stress that all play a role. Some people wake up one day and feel like a switch has been flipped and Energizer Bunny mode is on. Others observe a slow, gradual improvement in markers like energy and cravings, and still others need another week or two to adapt before the magic kicks in. If you haven't experienced Tiger Blood yet, it will come.

If you're not feeling Tiger Blood here are a few tips:

Eat More.

It's worth repeating. If you're active in your job, have a higher intensity workout routine and eating low-carb or low-fat, you are going to feel lethargic, and your performance will suffer. Adding more starchy carbs (like potatoes or winter squash) and fruit to each meal, and/or upping your fat intake, can flip things into high gear. Or, if you are overeating dried fruit, fruit-and-nut bars, or fruit smoothies/juices you may be sabotaging effective fat adaption by giving yourself sugar too often! Lean more on healthy fats and lower-carb veggies for a week and see if that does the trick.

Stop Grazing/Snacking.

If you're continuing to eat every 2-3 hours or consistently snacking/grazing between meals, you could be putting the brakes on your body learning how to generate steady, even energy. Your hormones need time between meals to do their job and let you tap into body and dietary fat for energy! If you are truly hungry between meals, immediately start making each meal bigger and continue doing that until three or four meals a day are doing the trick.

Stop comparing.

I am so blessed to be on this journey with you and grateful for this support group. I know I would have never been able to do this on my own but there may be one downfall to a support group like this and I want to nip it in the bud: comparing yourself to others. It could be the thief of your 30 Day Reset experience. Just because someone has gone down a pant size or is killing it in their workouts or has had some other NSVs doesn't mean you will have the same experience or that you are doing anything wrong. The timeline given, provides a general frame of reference for what most people experience along the way, but it's not a one-size fits-all- especially when it comes to Tiger Blood.

Stay focused on your own experience, enjoy the good things that are happening and embrace your own journey, wherever you are!

> "For I know the plans I have for you, declares the Lord, plans to prosper you and not to harm you, plans to give you hope and a future."
> Jeremiah 29:11

Reflect on how you have been successful these last 17 days? What changes have you noticed big or small? What are you hearing others say about you?

_____

_____

_____

_____

DAY EIGHTEEN

LET GO AND LET GOD.

Have you ever been so immersed in something it consumes your life? You just want control over this thing and you will do everything in your power to determine the outcome. I have and I'm sure I'm not alone. Maybe that's how you have been feeling on this 30 Day Reset Journey. For the past 18 days your life has revolved around food. It's consumed every aspect of your life from the moment you wake up in the morning until the time you go to bed. You are constantly thinking about what you're going to make for the next meal, how you're going to attend the next social event, grocery shopping, doing the dishes and the list goes on.

This morning in my daily Bible reading I was convicted of being consumed by something that ultimately is out of my control. It doesn't mean I sit back and do nothing, but it has become my "god" in a sense. So, what have I learned and what has God graciously revealed to me and wants me to share with you this morning? "Let go and Let God!"

What does this phrase mean?

"Let go and let God" is a phrase that popped up several years ago and is still used today. Nowhere in the Bible does it actually say, Let go and let God. It doesn't mean we sit back and do nothing, feel nothing and live allowing circumstances to move us wherever they may. Sitting back and watching events unfold without being intentional is not what letting go and letting God is all about. 1 Timothy 6:12 tells us to "Fight the good fight of faith. Take hold of the eternal life to which you were called and about which you made the good confession in the presence of many witnesses." To fight and take hold are action words. They require us to do something. In fact, to fight requires strategy, being intentional and being equipped if your desire is to win. Now that doesn't sound like letting go and letting God, does it?

Jesus spoke these words to his disciples, "I am the vine, you are the branches. Whoever abides in me and I in him, he it is that bears much fruit, for apart from me you can do nothing." John 15:5. Take in that last phrase. "Apart from me you can do nothing." We can do lots of "stuff" and assume we are doing it for God, but if we are doing it on our own power and giving ourselves the credit, we are not letting go and letting God.

Letting go and letting God does not mean we will go without struggles. "Count it all joy, my brothers, when you meet trials of various kinds, for you know that the testing of your faith produces steadfastness." James 1:2-3. In fact, God uses struggles to grow us in our faith, to mature us and make us stronger to handle the next one while we spend just a short time on this earth compared to eternity.

Letting go and letting God is this "And we know that for those who love God all things work together for good" Romans 8:28 and the result of letting go and letting God will be that "the peace of God, which transcends all understanding, will guard your heart and your minds in Jesus Christ." Philippians 4:7

In Christ, we can face the trials of life with grace and good humor and complete faith that whatever God has for us is ok.

My prayer for all of you today is that whatever struggle you are facing, whether it's this 30 Day Reset Journey or something else, that you not rely on your own power, that you Let Go and Let God.

What struggle are you needing to let go and let God handle for you?

_____

_____

_____

_____

Take a few minutes to talk to God and tell Him how you are feeling? Thank him for this journey and for the healthy body He has given you? Hand over your struggle to Him and allow Him to work all things out for your good and His glory!

DAY NINETEEN

LETS SPICE THINGS UP!

In 2018, I did my first round of Whole 30 and I found I got bored eating the same foods. This challenged me to go outside my comfort zone and try some new things. Curry became an exciting new add to my lifestyle. My family now enjoys an entirely new flavor of food and I want to share one of my recipes with you for you to enjoy as well:

Red Curry With Vegetables (30 Day Reset and Paleo)

Ingredients:
   3 Carrots
   2 Garlic Cloves
   1 tbsp fresh ginger
   1 orange, green, red or yellow pepper
   other veggies (broccoli, mushrooms, zucchini, asparagus, cauliflower, kale)
   1/2 white onion
   Cauliflower Rice (or regular rice if not going for Whole 30 compliant)
Canned Goods
   1 can Organic Coconut Milk
   4 tbsp Thai red curry paste
Condiments
   1 tbsp Coconut Aminos (Tamari or soy sauce if not going for Whole 30 compliant)
Banking Spices
   Salt and Pepper
Oils & Vinegars
   2 tbsp Coconut or Olive Oil
Optional: chicken, shrimp, beef, sausage or other meat

Instructions:

1. Warm a large skillet with deep sides over medium heat. Once it is hot, add the oil. Add the onion and sprinkle of salt and cook, stirring often, until the onion has softened and is turning translucent, about 5 minutes. Add the ginger and garlic and cook until fragrant, about 30 seconds, while stirring continuously.
2. Add the bell peppers, carrots and any other vegetables. Cook until the vegetables are tender (3-5 minutes) stirring occasionally. Then add the curry paste and cook, stirring often, for 2 minutes.
3. Add the coconut milk and water, stir to combine. Bring the mixture to a simmer over medium heat, Reduce heat as necessary to maintain a gentle simmer and cook until vegetables are softened to your liking, about 5-10 minutes, stirring occasionally.
4. While simmering, make your steamed cauliflower rice. I just use frozen!
5. Remove from heat and season with coconut aminos and salt, to taste.

Optional – you can also add shrimp, ground turkey, beef, steak for extra protein. I cook separately and add at step 3.

Check in.

Today's Non Scale Victories

Rate on a Scale of 1-10 with 1 being the worst and 10 being the best.

Energy

        Worst   1   2   3   4   5   6   7   8   9   10   Best

Sleep Quality

        Worst   1   2   3   4   5   6   7   8   9   10   Best

Cravings

        Worst   1   2   3   4   5   6   7   8   9   10   Best

DAY TWENTY

GOOD MORNING, RISE AND SHINE.

At this point in your 30 Day Reset journey you may be having Good Mornings indeed. You are falling asleep faster, your sleeping more deeply and waking up earlier, refreshed and energized. This is one of the coolest and most underrated 30 Day Reset NSV.

In todays overscheduled world, it's a badge of honor to be exhausted. We brag about how busy we are, how little we sleep and how hard we work. It feels lazy and selfish to go to bed early or take a nap, but I'm here to tell you sleep is an incredible resource. Not enough messes up basically everything, but better sleep can HELP mood, focus, energy and even weight loss. If you're finding some areas of sleep are better (falling asleep faster) but others are worse (waking more frequently) know this is normal as hormonal rhythms shift. Likely on this journey, your relationship with sleep and "busy-ness" is another thing you'll likely improve during your 30 days.

Favorite tricks for getting the best night's sleep:

Pre-bed habits.

The "blue lights" emanating from your smartphone, tablet or television are especially disruptive at night, suppressing melatonin secretion and messing with your sleep. Your best practice is to have zero screen-time in the hour before bed. Besides, You don't need to read unsettling information on Facebook/Twitter/Email right before you go to bed anyway. It's also ideal to finish all exercise sessions at least 3 hours before bed -especially high intensity activity, which can ramp up your cortisol production when they should be at their low.

Your bedtime environment.

Studies show you sleep best in a cool, dark room. Hang blackout curtains, remove or turn off all electronics and if you sleep with your phone in the room make sure it is on "airplane mode"

Establish a routine.

Setting a nightly routine can help your body know it's time for bed. Maybe is a bath with Epsom salt and peace and calming oil, meditation, prayer, reading a good book, a cup of herbal tea (Sleepy Time), gentle stretching or yoga, placing a diffuser in your bedroom and use lavender or cedarwood essential oil. Whatever you do, at the end of the day count your blessings and consciously forgive yourself and others for hurts accumulated during the day to unwind and prepare yourself for a good night's rest.

How can you improve the amount and quality of rest you are getting?

_____

_____

_____

_____

Do you struggle with being "busy"? What things could you cut out or say "No" to that may not align with your values, may be taking up too much time and causing conflict with your spouse or family. Take a few moments to reflect on your busyness.

_____

_____

_____

"For anyone who enters God's rest also rests from their works, just as God did from his."

Hebrews 4:10

DAY TWENTY-ONE

ONLY 9 DAYS LEFT.

Feeling nervous or excited today? Only 9 days left, and you are on your own. Only 9 more days and you've made it through the journey. The light at the end of this health and habit tunnel is just around the corner. You have thrived through three entire weekends and only have one more to go.

The food rut.

If you can't eat another egg if it was the last thing on the planet, or if nothing sounds good to you, you are in a food rut. It happens to most of us. I have met a few people that can eat the same thing every day for weeks. I admire them, but this is not me! I have to change things up and keep things exciting to keep myself motivated. Today is all about making sure your last 9 days are just as exciting as the first 9 days, minus the headaches, lethargy and Sugar Dragon.

Now that you have your pantry stocked with the essentials, food prep, meal planning and emergency foods are on autopilot, it's time to get a little creative in the kitchen and take your 30 Day Reset to the next level. This will also help prepare you for life after The 30 Day Reset for those planning to make this a permanent lifestyle change.

Try New Foods.

Eggs are easy, and avocado and sweet potato are delicious, but there are other protein, fat, and carb sources. Start by trying a new vegetable or two. Local farmers markets are a great place to score something fresh and get tips about how to prepare it.

New Seasonings.

Adding new seasonings and trying new seasoning mixtures can really spice things up. Don't be afraid. New and more seasonings really enhance the flavor of your food and make all the difference in a bland dish versus an exceptional dish you will be excited to make again.

New Recipes.

This is where you get the most bang for your buck. Discovering a new favorite dish (Curry for me) can energize your 30 Day Reset for days. Reaching out to someone with similar tastes or cooking preferences can make the recipe finding job easier. Use this group to ask and bounce ideas off one another. Be sure to check out my website www.lisamcquillen.com, Browse Pinterest, The Whole30 website or check out websites like Wellness Mama and PaleoRunningMomma.

My personal goal during this journey was to try one new recipe each week. If you try a new recipe every day you may be setting yourself up to fail and your family may go a little crazy. Find what works for you and don't make them complicated!

What new recipes are you going to try?

_____

_____

_____

_____

Add them to your meal planning sheet and choose days you won't be rushed or have plenty of time to enjoy being in the kitchen.

Check in.

Today's Non Scale Victories.

Rate on a Scale of 1-10 with 1 being the worst and 10 being the best.

Energy

       Worst   1   2   3   4   5   6   7   8   9   10   Best

Sleep Quality

       Worst   1   2   3   4   5   6   7   8   9   10   Best

Cravings

       Worst   1   2   3   4   5   6   7   8   9   10   Best

DAY TWENTY-TWO

GET MOVING.

Day 22 will have you feeling more inspired, energized and motivated. You've got this 30 Day Reset down and things are on cruise control. Add a little exercise into the mix. Play tag or kickball with your kids, or try something new like Tabata or Yoga. Sign up for your first 5K. The key to sticking with an exercise program is to change it up and make it fun.

Here is a list of ideas:

Brisk walking
Yoga
Dancing
Zumba
Bike ridding
Tennis
Downhill Skiing
Playing Baseball, Tag, Soccer or Kickball with your kids
Running
Swimming
Snow shoeing
Gardening
Hiking
Tabata
Cross Country Skiing
Kayaking or Paddle Boarding
Take your kids to a playground or on a fitness scavenger hunt

Using a Push Lawn Mower
Pickleball

What's the benefit, anyway?

Regular physical activity can improve your muscle strength and boost your endurance. Exercise delivers oxygen and nutrients to your tissues and helps your cardiovascular system work more efficiently, reducing your risk of chronic disease. Exercise increases the production of endorphins, which are known to help produce positive feelings and reduce the perception of pain, making you feel happier. Regular moderate exercise can increase your body's production of natural antioxidants, protecting your skin cells and delay signs of aging. Exercise can help you sleep better and feel more energized during the day.

I enjoy early morning runs or biking as a time to reflect, pray and prepare for the day! I recently tried Tabata and our family picked up tennis. What's your favorite way to get moving? What new activity or adventure could you add to the mix?

What is your favorite way to get moving? What new activity or adventure could you add to the mix?

_____

_____

_____

_____

_____

_____

DAY TWENTY-THREE

WHOLE 30 ON A BUDGET.

You will wake up today feeling your new 30 Day Reset normal—energized, happy, healthy and normal. You are not even thinking about being on the 30 Day Reset, you're just thinking, it feels so good! You are doing awesome and your hard work, commitment and discipline are paying off. About this time, the idea of continuing longer than 30 days doesn't seem so scary. This could be your new forever lifestyle, with a couple exceptions (an occasional glass of wine and piece of dark chocolate), but you are thinking it gets expensive eating like this and I'm constantly buying groceries.

Is It Really More Expensive?

My personal experience in the beginning was exactly what I mentioned above. I was surprised at how much we were spending on groceries. My husband and I do the Dave Ramsey cash envelope system and we had to increase our grocery envelope, but there were other areas we were spending less including going out to eat, alcohol, convenient store snacks while we were on the go and the biggest area was my husband's daily eating out while on the road. This alone saved us about $50 a week. I was no longer purchasing bags of chips, boxed cereals and boxes of processed crackers or snacks that add up in a hurry. Actually, there are aisles in the grocery store I haven't seen in months and it feels good. What also feels good is pulling up to the check-out counter with a cart loaded with fresh produce that I know will get consumed and not go to waste.

Meal Planning.

In the past I felt as though I was tossing a lot of old food out of the refrigerator.

Money down the garbage disposal. Meal Planning for the week and purchasing exactly what I need on my grocery list has cut down on this tremendously and in the long run savings money.

Grow your own.

For some, gardening is an option for eating fresh fruits and vegetables. Maybe it's time to try something new and start your own garden. Help a friend or neighbor and share the produce. Tomatoes and peppers are great to toss in the freezer for the winter months to make soups and sauces. Potatoes are a staple in my home and can last several months in a cool dark basement. Carrots, peas, raspberries, strawberries, apples, rhubarb, zucchini can all be frozen and used in later when you are bundled up inside on a cold blistery day (did I really just say that!?). Cucumbers to pickles, the list goes on of the possibilities. I have also found working in my garden to be a de-stressor and my son loves to help out (for a few more years anyway). There is so much to learn and teach your children through gardening!

Buy in Season.

If you don't have a green thumb to save your soul, explore this strategy. Local farmers markets are another great option and you can find great deals on in-season produce while also helping your local economy. This is also a great time to try something new. After all, if it's in season, you won't feel as bad if it is a flop. Yes, I've had a few meals that weren't masterpieces, but no one starved. As you shop the grocery store, look for in season produce which can be a huge break for your wallet. You can even stock up on these and toss them in the freezer for later.

Try Less Expensive Cuts of Meat.

Check the sales and stock up. Try chicken thighs instead of chicken breasts. Different cooking methods are also a great idea, like a slow cooker, to make tougher cuts of meat tender and juicy. You can also look for cheaper cuts that will yield leftovers such as a whole chicken, pork belly or shoulder.

How can you incorporate some of these suggestions to be more mindful of your resources and what recipes are you going to try?

_____

_____

_____

_____

What went well today?

_____

_____

_____

_____

DAY TWENTY-FOUR

ONE WEEK LEFT

Choose the mindset most closely resembling your experience right now. Are you thinking, "yes it's almost over" or are you thinking "I feel great and think I will keep going?"

The 30 Day Reset is just the first step in a lifelong journey of discovering your food freedom. You won't have to eat like this forever, and some of your old favorites MAY make the cut back into your regular healthy eating plan, but if you really want a healthy, sustainable, rewarding diet that will bring you a lifetime of benefits, you will have to continue practicing mindfulness, awareness and conscientiousness around food for the rest of your life. If you have been thinking about the 30 Day Reset "ending," reframe your focus. This is just the first step, and it only gets better.

Research around habits shows that when your brain perceives reward on the horizon, cravings come back with a vengeance. This partially explains why people binge hard after coming off a short-term weight loss diet. The diet is "over" and the brain wants everything you've been denying it, all at once. It is vital not to think about your 30 Day Reset as "ending", just transitioning into the next phase. If you are thinking about the end, tell your brain to "Calm down, nothing's over just yet. We are just going to keep rolling with all these amazing benefits and delicious, satisfying foods."

Commit to making your last week of 30 Day Reset the best one yet. For many, this last week brings even MORE magic, but only if you keep actively working the program.

How can you recommit and refocus today?

_____

_____

_____

_____

How are you feeling about making this a more permanent lifestyle? Have you talked to your family about what their thoughts are?

_____

_____

_____

_____

DAY TWENTY-FIVE

HAPPY DAY 25!

Your 30 Day Reset is bright and shiny again, and you're finally committed to finishing strong. In fact, you're feeling so good and things are going so well that you're wondering if you should make it a Whole40 or Whole60.

It's common for people to consider extending their program at this point in the journey. Between now and Day 30 it's common for people to think "I could do this forever" and "I can't wait to reintroduce." So, don't make any hasty decisions – you've got 5 more days to figure it out. In the meantime, enjoy your Tiger Blood, enjoy the encouragement from your 30 Day Reset group and see what additional benefits you can squeeze out of your 30 Day Reset.

There are a number of reasons you are considering extending your 30 Day Reset journey but being afraid to let go of the rules or eat something not-The 30 Day Reset isn't one of them. We have eliminated them because they are unknown (and often problematic). The 30 Day Reset experiment is designed to help you figure out how these foods work for you, so you can bring your choice of delicious, special or culturally-relevant foods back into your life in a way that works for you. Once and for all, experiencing Food Freedom.

How do I know if extending my 30 Day Reset or completing another 30 days is right for me?

Medical Conditions.

I am not a doctor, but through this journey I have learned to listen to my body. If you have a longstanding medical condition, especially chronic pain, fatigue, auto immune illness, stiffness, infertility for example, 30 days probably isn't long enough. My husband just told me last night that his heel pain is gone, and we've been doing this for 3 months. If you are already seeing some improvements, it might be a good indication that more time could bring you more results.

Food Addictions.

If you've had a long history with serious cravings or consider yourself a sugar or carb addict, you may want to stay on the 30 Day Reset until you feel totally in control and ready to reintroduce potentially triggering foods.

Stressful Events.

If you've got a stressful but short-term event during or just after Day 31, staying on the program through this time period can help you keep calm and focused. It reduces the risk that stress will drive you right back into old comfort habits.

Another unintended benefit many see is weight loss, however this is not the goal of the plan. If your goal is to continue to see improvements in this area or want to keep the extra pounds off you may want to consider extending.

To all the women in this group, (sorry guys).

Most of us are the gate keepers to the things that come in our home whether its food, cleaning products, personal care products, etc. We have the power to influence our families and the decisions our children will make when they get out on their own. We also have the power to influence their attitudes and the eternity of their souls.

What kind of influence do you want to have on your family, children, friends?

_____

_____

_____

_____

What is the long term impact continuing on this journey could have on you, your family, your children and those around you?

_____

_____

_____

_____

"She is clothed with strength and dignity and she laughs without fear of the future. When she speaks, her words are wise, and she gives instructions with kindness. She carefully watches everything in her household and suffers nothing from laziness"

Proverbs 31:25-31

26

DAY TWENTY-SIX

A NEW PERSPECTIVE

By now you have noticed you have a new perspective on life. You are less anxious or calmer in general. You find yourself being in the moment more with your husband, children, co-workers, etc. You handle stress more gracefully. You're able to focus better, are more productive and creative. Maybe you're trying new things you've always wanted to try, you are engaging with the world!

Organic Foods.

This morning I would like to share with you a new perspective on organic foods. I was raised on a family farm that produced corn and beans. We also raised beef cattle and hogs. I fully respect with gratitude, the hard work, sacrifices and dedication it takes to be a farmer and help feed the world. This by no means is a bash on non-organic farmers. It is worth noting, we do not consume 100% organic in my household. If I have the option and I feel it fits within our budget, I will choose organic. But I currently have a freezer full of meat raised by my nephews and I don't plan on changing that anytime soon. I have transitioned to 100% all-natural cleaning and personal care products through Young Living. Let me know, I would love to share more about this lifestyle with you. You can connect with me on Facebook, Instagram or by emailing me at mcquillen14@gmail.com

3 Reason Organic Matters To Me:

They are better for us.

Organic doesn't necessarily mean the foods are more nutritious, but it does mean they are inherently less harmful because of their decreased exposure to chemicals and pesticides. Chemicals and pesticides contain toxins and heavy metals that affect our bodies at a cellular level and disrupt our hormones and can take a toll on our joints, muscles and major organs over time.

It's good for the environment and for the ecosystem.

It takes us back to where it all began – God! (My favorite reason).

In the beginning God created. You may remember how the story goes from one of the first chapters. Light, Dark, Clouds, Ocean, Sun, Moon, Stars and then Plants, Trees, Fruits and Vegetables. Fast forward several hundred or maybe even thousands of years later and God spoke to the Israelites. Remember this group of people? They were the same ones grumbling and complaining over food.

This group of people was just like you and me. They wanted to be in control, they wanted things to make them happy and comfortable, they wanted the easy way, not the narrow and more difficult path, so God had to give them lots of rules to protect them. Protect them from harm, from disease so they wouldn't die and many other issues.

The book of Leviticus is all about God's rules for these people to keep them safe so they could eventually get to the Promise Land. After all, they faced many obstacles while wandering in the wilderness for 40 years without the comforts we have today. Here is what I want to bring your attention to. In Leviticus 19:19 God said (thru Moses): "You shall keep my statutes. You shall not let your cattle breed with a different kind. You shall not sow your field with two kinds of seed, nor shall you wear a garment of cloth made of two kinds of material."

God commanded this to protect the Israelites and for their best interest to keep them pure and holy as they traveled to the promise land. God wants the same for us. He desires our souls to be pure and holy (with His food) so that one day when we meet him face to face He can welcome us home for eternity into the place He has been preparing for us.

The Environmental Working Group has a great "Dirty Dozen" guide to organics, which lists the fruits and vegetables most impacted by chemicals. On the flip side, the fruits and veggies in the "Clean 15" absorb a minimal amount of pesticides and fertilizers so there is little discrepancy between organic and conventional.

How can you be more open to other's perspectives?

_____

_____

_____

_____

What went well today?

_____

_____

_____

_____

What NSV are you experiencing?

_____

_____

_____

_____

DAY TWENTY-SEVEN

COOKING IT UP WITH LISA.

These tender grilled or baked pork chops are a family favorite. The marinade can also be used on chicken or steak. I like to serve these with mashed potatoes and green beans.

Tender Pork Chops

Ingredients:

> 4 boneless Pork loin Chops
> ¼ cup olive oil
> 2 ½ Tablespoons of Coconut Aminos
> 2 Tablespoons Homemade Montreal Steak Seasoning

Instructions:

Mix oil, Coconut Aminos and seasoning in small bowl and mix together.

Place the pork chops in a gallon zip lock bag and add seasoning mixture.

Refrigerate and marinade for 3-24 hours.

Montreal Steak Seasoning

Ingredients:

> 2 Tablespoons Paprika

> 2 Tablespoons freshly ground black pepper

1 Tablespoon kosher/coarse salt

1 Tablespoon garlic powder

1 Tablespoon onion powder

1 Tablespoon coriander

1 Tablespoon Dill

½ Tablespoon crushed red pepper flakes

Instructions:

Mix all the spices together and store in an airtight container. This will make a large batch that you will have prepared and ready to go for the next time!

Lemon Butter Green Beans

This has got to be one of the easiest recipes I've ever made and I'm quite embarrassed to say that this was my first time using fresh green beans and I will never go back. The taste, flavor and texture are so good, not to mention the nutritional benefits of fresh produce over canned or frozen. My only excuse for not cooking with fresh green beans before this was a lack of knowledge. I didn't know how, the best way to cook them, what seasonings to use. My lack of knowledge prevented me from enjoying a delicious vegetable in an entirely new way. I was sharing a few recipes with my Young Living family leading up to Thanksgiving and this one caught my eye. I decided to give it a try and you can too.

Ingredients:

1 pint fresh organic green beans (trim stem ends)
1 Tablespoon Salt
1 Tablespoons organic butter or ghee
1-2 drops of lemon vitality essential oil
Salt and Pepper to taste
Slivered almonds or cashews (optional)

Instructions:

Fill a medium sauce pan there quarters full of cold water.

Set over high heat and bring to a boil.

Add salt and 1 pint of fresh, organic if possible, green beans (washed and ends cut off).

Cook until water returns to a boil and beans are tender, about 5 minutes, Remove from heat and drain.

Immediately return the beans to saucepan.

Add 2 Tablespoons of organic butter or ghee and 1-2 drops of lemon vitality oil.

Add slivered almonds or cashews (optional).

Toss and season with salt and pepper.

Mashed Potatoes

Ingredients:

6-8 medium potatoes
Organic butter or ghee
1 can Organic Coconut Milk

Instructions:

Bring a pan water in a double broiler to a boil

Clean and peel potatoes. Cut into 1-2 inch sections and place in the top of double broiler for 10-15 minutes or until potatoes are soft and break apart.

Place potatoes in a mixing bowl. Add 2 tablespoons of organic butter or ghee and organic coconut milk.

Season with salt and pepper.

Blend with a hand mixer until you have the desired consistency. You may not need to use all of the coconut milk.

DAY TWENTY-EIGHT

GOOD MORNING

You look and feel awesome. Life is good. Perhaps you are a little nervous and even fearful of approaching Day 31. What if I fall back into my old habits, what if my asthma or allergies return, am I going to cave at every social function, is there a holiday coming up you are worried about? Will reintroducing foods deplete my Tiger Blood? We will be covering reintroduction tomorrow and Wednesday. Don't worry, you will be just fine.

Handling fear and worry.

We are a society filled with Fear and Worry. Recently I listened to a sermon on fear and worry titled "I worry something bad might happen." Some of you are saying right now, well of course that's my job as a parent or spouse or whatever role you play. I'm pretty sure every single one of us has experienced worry keeping us up at night.

So often when we are going through a valley or season of trials and tribulations we don't see what's right in front of us and the blessings that come from going through these experiences. We were asked to rate ourselves on a scaled of 1-10 on how well we see the goodness of God in our lives. I am challenging you to do the same right now.

Rate yourself on a scale of 1-10 with 1 being no fear or worry and 10 being, very fearful, anxiety, can't sleep fear and worry.

Fear

        Best   1 2 3 4 5 6 7 8 9 10 Worst

Worry

        Best   1 2 3 4 5 6 7 8 9 10 Worst

A little more about fear.

F - False

E - Evidence

A - About

R – Reality

Are you a half glass empty or half glass full kind of person? Do you tend to see the positives in life or are you quick to point out the negatives? Do people refer to you as a "Negative Nelly" or "Realist"? I'm not saying it's not ok to point out the obvious or talk about the facts. Examine the lens are you viewing your life right now. Through God's eyes and the blessings which He has poured out on you or through your own eyes and all the things that are going wrong?

Most of us tend to do the latter, which results in us worrying about something bad happening to us in the future.

Shift your mindset.

I'm challenging you to shift your mindset as we draw near to the end of this journey. If you rated yourself a 2, 5 or 7 on the scale. Take your mindset one number higher. It takes effort but it is worth it.

> "Finally, brothers, whatever is true, whatever is honorable, whatever is just, whatever is pure, whatever is lovely, whatever is commendable, if there is any excellence, if there is anything worthy of praise, think about these things."

> Philippians 4:8

You have to train your mind to think about these things. And ask for help. What if for the next 7 days you made an effort to focus on one of these things, such as what is honorable in your spouse or what is lovely in your children?

Write them down, tell them and thank God for them. I bet you would see a difference in your relationships and likely a shift in your thoughts.

_____

_____

_____

_____

As we approach Day 31, focus on God's blessings in your life, finish strong and grateful for the work that has been done in the last 30 days. Choose a positive mind and a positive life.

> "Run with endurance the race that has been set before us, looking to Jesus, the founder and perfecter of our faith, who for the joy that as set before him endured the cross, despising the shame, and is seated at the right hand of the throne of God"
>
> Hebrews 12:1

DAY TWENTY-NINE

WHAT'S NEXT?

You've got one day left and you are bound and determined to cruise through these next 24 hours with ease and confidence. In fact, you may be feeling more self-confident than ever knowing that you have battled through the cravings, naps, temptations, highs and lows to get to how awesome you are feeling today.

This is called Food Freedom. You are feeling in control of your food choices for the first time in your life. You have been disciplined and determined to make these positive changes in your life and in the life of your family. I believe all good things take commitment, dedication, and obedience. Healthy relationships, financial freedom, raising children, getting an education, spirituality and the list goes on. I believe wellness falls into this category. If it were easy, everyone would be doing it.

> "No discipline seems pleasant at the time, but painful. Later on, however, it produces a harvest of righteousness and peace for those who have been trained by it."
> Hebrews 12:11

> "Whoever heeds discipline shows the way of life, but whoever ignores correction leads others astray"
> Proverbs 10:17

> "Whoever loves discipline loves knowledge, but whoever hates correction is stupid."
> Proverbs 12:1

Some of you may still be looking for more results. More NSV and if you have been battling something chronic for a long time, 30 days may not be long enough for you. You may want to considering going another 30 days before reintroducing other foods. This is where you get to be in control and decide what's best for you. 30 Day Reset is not a one size fits all.

What does life after The 30 Day Reset look like for you? How can you find balance and remain confident in this new lifestyle you have discovered?

_____

_____

_____

_____

_____

_____

_____

DAY THIRTY

IT'S HERE, IT'S HERE, DAY 30!

You did it and I couldn't be happier or more proud of you. You feel amazing, you can't stop grinning and you just want to shout out to the entire world "I did it, I finished the 30 Day Reset!"

Take a second and celebrate.

Conquering it.

You took on something that you knew would be hard and you worked on it every single day, with purpose and determination. You experience plenty of challenges – some that made you wonder if you should just give up. Still, you persevered! You struggled physically and emotionally in the beginning, remember those days? It took sheer willpower, maybe a little stubbornness and prayer for some to get through a few of those days.

Finishing with abundance.

Remember this feeling. Savor it, reflect on it, journal about it. The next time life gets rough (and I promise it will), remember this journey, taking on something you didn't think you could accomplish and you didn't give up. You are celebrating tonight with a glass of wine or maybe you will find a new way to celebrate that doesn't revolve around food. You host a party serving a 30 Day Reset approved menu. Your success may just inspire the next person to change their lives and the lives of their children forever.

Tell me about it.

I want to hear your successes and join in your celebration. I want to experience your joy and encourage you in whatever your next phase, whatever that might be. I want to hear from you. Your energy, enthusiasm and happiness will be contagious and inspire others to change their lives too. Share your success with my at mcquillen14@gmail.com

Reflection on the past 30 days.

_____

_____

_____

_____

_____

_____

_____

_____

_____

_____

_____

_____

_____

_____

_____

The Fast Track Reintroduction.

I don't want to steal your thunder and excitement for today, but I also want you to be prepared for the reintroduction phase. I'm choosing to share with you the Fast Track Reintroduction. If you would like more information on the Slow Roll Reintroduction, contact me and I will get you the info.

Three keys to a successful 30 Day Reset Reintroductions:

1- Do not rush the process
2- Commit to self-awareness
3- Journal and take good notes

These are the areas you want to pay attention to: Digestion, Energy, Sleep, Cravings, Mood and Psychology, Behavior, Skin, Breathing, Pain/Inflammation, Medical Conditions/Symptoms.

Here is how it works. The Fast Track Reintroduction Schedule is designed to expose you to all previously eliminated food groups in 10-14 days, in order of least likely to most likely be problematic.

Sample Schedule

Day 1 (Optional): Evaluate gluten-free alcohol, while keeping the rest of your diet 30 Day Reset compliant.

Day 1 (OR 4): Evaluate legumes, while keeping the rest of your diet 30 Day Reset compliant. Ex. Peanut butter, edamame or tofu, black beans, hummus

Day 4 (OR 7): Evaluate non-gluten grains, while keeping the rest of your diet 30 Day Reset compliant. Ex. Gluten-free oats, rice, 100% corn tortillas, gluten-free bread, quinoa, etc.

Day 7 (OR 10): Evaluate dairy, while keeping the rest of your diet 30 Day Reset compliant. Ex. Plain (unsweetened) yogurt, milk or cream, cheese, sour cream

Day 10 (OR 13): Evaluate gluten-containing grains, while keeping the rest of your diet 30 Day Reset compliant. Ex. Whole wheat cereal, bread, crackers, pasta, beer

Day 1 Food Group

_____

_____

Reintroduced Foods

_____

_____

Observations

_____

_____

Day 4 Food Group

_____

_____

Reintroduced Foods

_____

_____

Observations

_____

_____

Day 7 Food Group

_____

_____

Reintroduced Foods

_____

_____

Observations

_____

_____

Day 10 Food Group

_____

_____

Reintroduced Foods

_____

_____

Observations

_____

_____

Day 13 Food Group

_____

_____

Reintroduced Foods

_____

_____

Observations

_____

_____

Hear what I have experienced and observed.

We have been reintroducing foods over the past couple weeks and here are some of the observations we have made:

- Cheese is not our friend! It does not agree with our digestive system.

- Sugar robs our energy.

- For me personally, I do ok with gluten free alcohol (Titos), but anything else makes me feel sluggish the next day!

- We have not yet reintroduced grains other than I made a pizza with a gluten free crust. I don't know if it was the crust or the cheese, but it did not agree with either one of us. I couldn't sleep that night and we both had unexpected trips to the bathroom.

- We have both learned to listen to our bodies and know when we have gone too far with foods that don't agree with our bodies. I believe this to be our biggest success. We are quickly eager to get back on track and be diligent about consuming real foods.

APPENDIX A

DO'S AND DON'TS FOR THE NEXT 30 DAYS

Do not consume sugar or added sugar of any kind! It doesn't matter if it is real or artificial. Here is a list (not inclusive, but a good start): Barley malt, Cane sugar (even if it says organic), Corn Syrup, evaporated cane juice, fruit juice, fructose, galactose, glucose, high fructose corn syrup, lactose, maltose, maltodextrin, mannitol, sucrose, sorbitol. Other sweeteners include coconut sugar, raw honey, date sugar, luo han guo (monk fruit), stevia, maple syrup, Xylitol.

Do not consume alcohol in any form. Not even a splash for cooking! No wine, beer, champagne, vodka, run, whiskey, tequila, etc.

Do not eat grains of any kind. This is more than gluten free. No wheat, rye, barley, oats, corn, rice, millet, bulgur, sorghum, sprouted grains, and all gluten free alternatives. Read your labels! Corn and wheat are added into so many of our foods in the form of bran, germ, starch, etc.

Do not eat legumes. This includes beans of all kinds with the exception of green beans, snow peas and sugar snap peas. Otherwise beans weather they are black, red, pinto, navy, white, kidney, lima, fava are off limits. Also peas, chickpeas, lentils and peanuts are not edible for the next 30 days. This includes no peanut butter (try almond butter), all forms of soy (soy sauce, miso, tofu, tempeh, edamame and any other foods that have soy snuck into them. You'll be surprised! Read your labels!

Do not eat dairy. This includes cow and goat milk as well as cream, cheese, kefir, yogurt and sour cream. The only exception to this rule is clarified butter or ghee.

Do not consume Carrageenan, MSG, or added Sulfites. Check the ingredients and read your labels.

Do not recreate baked goods, treats or junk food. No coconut milk ice cream, banana muffins, almond flour pancakes, Paleo bread, etc. Your cravings and habits won't be allowed to change if you keep feeding your body these foods.

Do not step on the scale or take measurements other than on day 1! This is not about counting calories or weight loss. There are so many bigger and better benefits to this journey than a number. You have to just trust me on this one!

Organic Fruit Juices are permitted, however, don't go overboard or rely on this to fix a craving you are having.

Most forms of vinegar are allowed with the exception of flavored vinegars with added sugar. White vinegar, balsamic, apple cider, red wine, white wine, champagne and rice vinegar are allowed as long as there is no added sugars.

Eat all the meat, seafood, eggs, vegetables, fruit and natural fats you can handle. You should not go hungry! You can tweak this along the way if you are looking for additional weight loss goals, but that should not be your primary focus at the beginning.

ABOUT THE AUTHOR

A wife, a mother, a sister, a daughter, an aunt, an employee, a co-worker, a friend and a follower of Jesus Christ. Wellness has always been at the core of who I am. My passion is helping others by empowering them to make choices that can change their life and the lives of future generations. By discovering pure wellness you will have the ability to find (or experience) joy, peace and freedom you have never experienced before.

In January of 2015, I attended a Young Living Essential Oils 101 Class that opened my eyes to a new world of wellness. Since then, God has blessed me with an abundance of opportunities to deepen my passion and has placed several amazing women in my life that have impacted my journey. My family (husband Mitch and 12 year old son Vince) are very active and love spending time in God's creation walking in the timber, gardening, hunting, fishing, running, boating and anything else that involves sports or the outdoors. I am always looking for ways to experience new adventures that continue to allow us to function the way our Creator made us.

Wherever you are at on your wellness journey or whatever your dreams may be, I am here to help you achieve abundance, purpose and wellness!

Made in the USA
San Bernardino, CA
02 January 2020